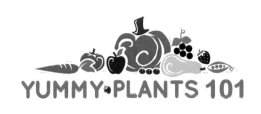

YUMMY·PLANTS 101

IT'S EASY

TO START EATING

VEGAN

REBECCA GILBERT

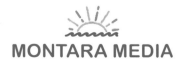

MONTARA MEDIA

"If you wanted to take advantage of the incredible benefits of a vegan diet but were not quite sure where to start, this is it! This easy, step-by-step guide brings you everything you need. This book is fun, authoritative, and written by someone who's made the transition you're about to make now. You will love it."

Neal D. Barnard, MD
President, Physicians Committee for
Responsible Medicine

"*Yummy Plants* is exactly what you can expect from Rebecca's book. This guide is filled with mouth-watering vegan recipes that will have your whole family asking for seconds. Get started on a healthier lifestyle right here!"

Robert Cheeke
Bestselling author of *Vegan Bodybuilding & Fitness –*
The Complete Guide to Building Your Body
on a Plant-Based Diet

"If you're on the fence about going vegan, read this book! You'll want to jump right in. Rebecca teaches you how to stock your vegan pantry so that you can start creating amazing meals in no time!"

Jenny Engel and Heather Goldberg
Co-Owners of Spork Foods

"She makes vegan food so accessible and irresistibly appealing to the millions of Americans who have never considered how delicious and beautiful a vegan diet can be."

Ellen Jaffe Jones, @vegcoach.com
Author of *Eat Vegan on $4 a Day, Kitchen Divided*,
and co-author of *Paleo Vegan*

"Demystifying the vegan diet with tips, charts, recipes, and explanations of all those weird grains you never heard of, *It's Easy to Start Eating Vegan! YUMMY PLANTS 101* is an easy to digest, nuts and bolts guide that I wish I had when I became vegan."

Brian L. Patton
Creator of thesexyvegan.com, and author of *The Sexy Vegan Cookbook* and *The Sexy Vegan's Happy Hour at Home*

"Making delicious plant-based recipes accessible to everyone is an important step in saving our health, the animals and the environment, and Rebecca Gilbert's excellent new book makes it easy to start eating vegan! Chock full of basic tips, helpful lists, sample meal plans and super yummy recipes, this book is a must read for anyone who is looking to adopt a vegan lifestyle!"

Laura Theodore
Host of the PBS vegan cooking series *Jazzy Vegetarian*,
and author of *Jazzy Vegetarian Classics*

It's Easy to Start Eating Vegan! YUMMY PLANTS® 101
Published by Montara Media, LLC
Copyright © 2014 Rebecca Gilbert

ISBN: 9780990395706

Library of Congress Control Number: 2014940317

10 9 8 7 6 5 4 3 2 1

Company products/ brand names have been listed to help readers find vegan products in grocery stores or online. Author has not received any compensation for mentioning company products/ brand names or including coupons.

Author is not making any recommendations regarding specific products. All products represent that they meet all requirements to be labeled as vegan at the time of this printing.

Cover design: Marcy Smith
Illustrations: Marcy Smith
Interior layout and design: Jennifer A. Kambas
Photography: Neeti Attwood, Sushma Patel Bould, Greg Stratton

Printed in the United States of America
Printed on recycled paper ♻

For Ines, Kathrin, and Kristin

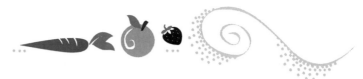

You have the power to create positive change in this world. It's time. Let's get started!

Rebecca Gilbert

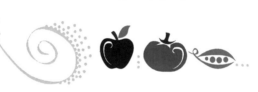

TABLE OF CONTENTS

INTRODUCTION

It's Easy to Start Eating Vegan!
YUMMY PLANTS 101

I wrote this guide to share what worked for me when I became vegan, so that when *you* decide to make the change, your journey will be easy and delicious.

Why did I choose to become a vegan? I wanted to improve my health, and I believed that changing what I ate could help me heal.

I was a former competitive figure skater. In my early 20s, my skating career ended because of severe, chronic joint pain. I could hardly walk! It was devastating. Not only was I brokenhearted about not being able to skate, but I couldn't even do normal things like walking up and down stairs. I lived on pain medication. It was awful.

Fast forward five years: I read about a Scandinavian study that suggested a vegan diet could reduce inflammation and eliminate chronic joint pain. The experimental group went vegan for six months and reported a significant reduction in their osteo-arthritic knee pain.

That was all I needed to hear. The next day I went vegan. Cold Tofurky.

I didn't know what I was doing, or that such things as egg replacers and dairy substitutions even existed. But I did know I wanted my life back. If switching to vegan food would heal me, I was committed to making the change.

After three weeks of eating purely plant-based nutrition, I was feeling much better. After five weeks, I returned to the ice. I was amazed. When I stopped eating animal products, the chronic joint pain I'd suffered for five years simply disappeared. I wish someone had told me about this earlier!

There are so many wonderful reasons to shift toward plant-based eating: for our health, for the environment, and for the animals. Although I became a vegan for health reasons, I now believe that animals are friends, not food.

I've been vegan for many years now, and I'm here to make the journey easy for you.

Are you ready to start a new adventure that offers endless benefits? If so, there are delicious, healthy, fulfilling vegan foods waiting for you!

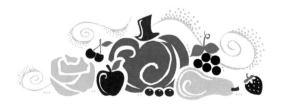

You can learn more about my story and
watch me start to skate again at:

▶ bit.ly/1mrmT8N

I was so grateful to get back on the ice!

Why Choose to Start Eating Vegan?

 It's good for your health. A plant-based diet can reverse heart disease, type 2 diabetes, and obesity.

 It's good for the environment. It reduces our carbon footprint.

 It's good for our resources. We can feed more people using the same arable land.

 It's absolutely good for the animals. We can meet all our nutritional needs from the plant kingdom.

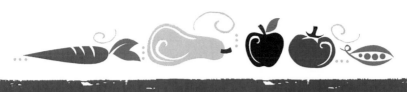

CHAPTER 1

Basics of a Vegan Diet

Many people think that being vegan means eating salads for breakfast, lunch, and dinner. Salads are definitely delicious, but they represent just a fraction of what we eat!

Like everyone else, we enjoy a wide variety of foods spanning the global spectrum, from pizza Margherita and French onion soup to spicy Asian stir-fries and Mexican burritos. We also indulge in ice-cream cones, holiday cookies, and even Halloween candy! The only difference is that in place of the meat, dairy, and other ingredients derived from animals, we choose foods made with healthier, cholesterol-free substitutes.

A great first step on your path towards eating vegan is to learn about plant-based protein sources and easy substitutions for eggs and dairy.

Vegan Dairy

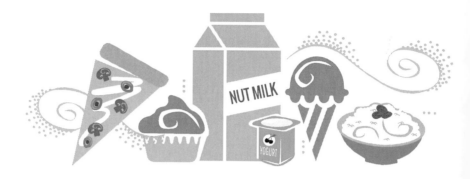

As a vegan, you can still enjoy your *café au lait*, cereal, and buttered toast for breakfast. It's just that the products you'll be using will be made from plants. Vegan "dairy" products are often made from oats, rice, flax seeds, soy, sunflower seeds, coconut, hemp, cashews, and almonds.

So, how do these plant-based products taste? Delicious! The milks are creamy, the butter is rich and spreadable. Is anything missing? Only the cholesterol!

Just like traditional dairy milks, there are vegan milks which are sold in both the refrigerated section of the grocery store and in the unrefrigerated drinks aisle. It's great to have shelf-stable mini milks on hand for lunches, picnics, or travel.

Yogurt – Yummy Probiotics

The beneficial bacteria found in traditional yogurts and keffirs are also found in vegan yogurts and keffirs made from coconut, almond, and soy milks. Common brands include So Delicious Dairy Free and Stonyfield O'Soy.

Summer Ice Cream Dreams

Ice cream can help you beat the summer heat. You'll find non-dairy ice cream and frozen novelties made from coconut milk, almond milk, rice milk, and soymilk. Common brands include Coconut Bliss, Rice Dream, So Delicious Dairy Free, and Tofutti. There is even a brand of raw vegan ice cream, Cashewtopia, which is made from cashew nuts.

Pizza, Anyone?

Vegan cheese is becoming so common that you'll find vegan pizzas in your supermarket's freezer section. (Try Amy's Organics or Daiya.) Making your own vegan pizza at home is another tasty option. Common cheese brands that really melt include Daiya, Follow Your Heart, Go Veggie, and Teese Cheese.

**Learn more about vegan dairy options
with this video on YouTube!**
▶ **bit.ly/1m3noV8**

In 2012, the Harvard School of Public Health published information that dairy is not the only nor the best source of calcium.[1]

Why?

1. Our bodies absorb plant-based calcium better than dairy-based calcium.

2. Plant-based calcium sources are cholesterol-free.

So where can we get our calcium? Plant-based calcium-rich alternatives include bok choy, broccoli, collards, kale, tofu, and baked beans.

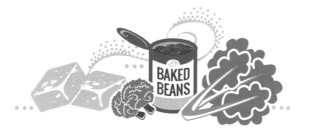

[1] *The Nutrition Source: Calcium and Milk*, Harvard School of Public Health www.hsph.harvard.edu/nutritionsource/ what-should-you-eat/calcium-and-milk/

What is casein?

Casein is a milk protein. People who suffer an inflammatory response to dairy products, who have symptoms like migraine headaches or chronic joint pain, may be affected by casein. Surprisingly, some "non-dairy" items do contain casein, including some otherwise vegan cheeses and yogurts. Companies sometimes take rice, soy, or almond products and add casein for creaminess. Luckily, it is possible to have vegan cheese that melts and yogurt that tastes creamy without casein. If you don't see "vegan" on the package, check the label to confirm casein isn't one of the ingredients.

Make your own nut milk at home!

Fresh nut milks are delicious and simple to prepare. You'll just need 2 cups of water and 1 cup of dry nuts. There are 3 basic steps: measure, soak, and blend.

1 Measure one cup of nuts and cover with water.

2 Soak according to the time chart below. Then discard soak water and rinse with fresh water.

3 Blend: Add 2 cups of water and process until smooth with a high powered blender like a Vitamix or Blendtec.

Note: If you want perfectly smooth nut milk, process longer or strain using a mesh nut milk bag.

During the processing, you can add optional flavoring like fresh vanilla bean, raw cacao nibs, or dates for sweetness.

Try a Vitamix with **free shipping**, visit **bit.ly/1nuTjEJ**

NUT	SOAK TIME
Almond	8-12 hours (overnight)
Brazil	no soaking required
Cashew	1-2 hours
Hazelnuts	no soaking required
Macadamia	no soaking required
Pecans	4-6 hours
Walnuts	4 hours

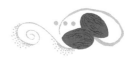

Eliminating Eggs

Tofu is a popular substitute for scrambled eggs, but it's not the best binder or raising agent for cooking and baking. There are many excellent egg replacers you can use when making cakes, cookies, and other baked goods.

Each of these substitutions is equal to one egg:

✓ 1 Tbsp. apple cider vinegar + 1 tsp. baking soda –
Works best as a **raising agent** for breads, cakes, and muffins

✓ ¼ cup apple sauce –
Works best a **binder** for cakes, muffins, and brownies

✓ ½ to 1 banana –
Works best as a **binder** for muffins and heavier baked goods like brownies

✓ 2 Tbsp. finely ground flax seed + 3 Tbsp. water –
Works best as a **binder** for cookies, cakes, and other baked goods

✓ 1½ Tbsp. Ener-G powdered egg replacer + 2 Tbsp. water –
Works as both a **binder** and **raising agent** in baked goods

Plant-Based Protein

While protein needs vary by individual activity levels, the CDC guidelines suggest that the average adult needs between 46g – 56g of protein per day. [2]

Athletes do have higher daily protein needs. However, weekend warriors and professional athletes alike can get more than enough protein each day from 100% plant-based sources. This sample menu from the Vegetarian Resource Group demonstrates the abundance and variety of vegan protein sources.

Breakfast: 1 cup oatmeal (6g)
1 cup soy milk (7g)
1 bagel (9g)
= 22g

Lunch: 2 slices whole wheat bread (5g)
1 cup vg baked beans (12g)
= 17g

Dinner: 5 oz. firm tofu (11g)
1 cup cooked broccoli (4g)
1 cup cooked brown rice (5g)
2 tablespoons almonds (4g)
= 24g

Snack: 2 tablespoons peanut butter (8g)
6 crackers (2g)
= 8g

Total = 73g of protein!

[2] www.cdc.gov/nutrition/everyone/basics/protein.html

Vegan Protein Powders

Supplements are another option to meet daily protein requirements. There are many brands available online or in vegan-friendly grocery stores. Look for products that are based on whole foods rather than food isolates.

How much protein do I need?

The Recommended Dietary Allowances (RDA) for different age groups are (*Source: CDC*):

RECOMMENDED DIETARY ALLOWANCE FOR PROTEIN	GRAMS OF PROTEIN NEEDED EACH DAY
Children ages 1 – 3	13
Children ages 4 – 8	19
Children ages 9 – 13	34
Girls ages 14 – 18	46
Boys ages 14 – 18	52
Women ages 19 – 70+	46
Men ages 19 – 70+	56

All fruits, vegetables, grains, and legumes contain protein. Plant-based protein sources don't contain any cholesterol!

Learn more about vegan protein sources!
▶ bit.ly/1jhzm2M

TOP 10 PLANT-BASED SOURCES OF PROTEIN

(See the entire list in the Appendix*)

Approximate protein per cup (cooked)

Soybeans	29g
Lentils	18g
Adzuki beans	17g
Split peas	16g
Black beans	15g
Chickpeas	15g
Great northern beans	15g
Kidney beans	15g
Lima beans	15g
Navy beans	15g

*See the Appendix starting on page 87
for a complete list of all plant-based proteins.

NOTABLE NUTS & SEEDS!

Nuts and seeds are loaded with protein. Sprinkle a handful on yogurt, salad, or fruit to boost the protein content.

Approximate protein per 1 oz

Pumpkin seeds	8g
Roasted peanuts	7g
Almonds	6g
Pistashios	6g
Cashews (raw)	5g
Sunflower seeds	5g
Brazil nuts	4g
Hazelnuts	4g
Walnuts	4g
Pecans	3g
Macadamia nuts	2g

Approximate protein per 1 Tbsp

Hemp seeds*	3g
Flaxseed	2g
Sesame seeds	2g

* Hemp seeds do not contain THC.

CHAPTER 2

Stock Your Vegan Fridge and Pantry

While it's key to eat fresh fruits and veggies, it's also a smart idea to have a supply of canned beans or frozen vegetables on hand for those nights when you want to whip up something nutritious and delicious in a hurry.

Perishable Basics

☐ Fresh fruits, vegetables, sprouts

☐ Vegan milk, creamer, yogurt, ice cream

☐ Vegan butter, cheese, cream cheese, sour cream, whipped cream

☐ Hummus (Try making your own! See page 75)

☐ Mock meats (that taste like chicken, bacon, and beef)

The Non-Perishable Basics

❑   Frozen vegetables: peas, broccoli, spinach, carrots

❑   Canned beans: black, pinto, kidney

❑   Dry beans, lentils, grains (See the Appendix, page 87, for an extensive list of grains.)

❑   Shelf-stable, non-dairy milk

❑   Egg replacer powder, apple cider vinegar, flax seeds, applesauce

❑   Frozen fruit for desserts or smoothies

❑   Vegan bouillon cubes

❑   Vegan sugar

❑   Cooking and baking oils such as olive oil and vegetable oil

❑   Nuts: almonds, cashews, peanuts, pecans, walnuts, pistachios

❑   Nut butters: peanut, almond, cashew

❑   Crunchy toppings: flax seeds, hemp seeds, chia seeds, cacao nibs

❑   Nutritional yeast: Tastes like cheese – sprinkle on salads, potatoes, beans, etc

❑   Vitamin B12

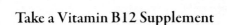

Take a Vitamin B12 Supplement

According to the Physicians
Committee for Responsible Medicine
(PCRM), vegans should take a
Vitamin B12 supplement. PCRM
says, "Overall, vegan diets provide
better nutrition than any other kind
of diet—with plenty of protein,
calcium, and iron, and an abundance
of vitamins and minerals—without
the problems posed by animal fat
and cholesterol. But it's essential to
include a source of vitamin B12."
And it's so easy. You can get B12
from a daily multiple vitamin or
B12 supplement, or fortified foods
(e.g., fortified cereals, soymilk, etc.).

*See your health care practitioner
for details and dosage amounts.*

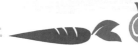

Common Brands

Vegan Dairy

Butter: Earth Balance, Nutiva, Spectrum (shortening, for baking)

Sour cream and cream cheese: Follow Your Heart, Tofutti

Mayonaise: Earth Balance, Just Mayo, Vegenaise

Ice cream: Almond Dream, Cashewtopia, Coconut Bliss, Rice Dream, So Delicious Dairy Free, Tofutti

Cheese: Daiya, Follow Your Heart, Go Veggie, Kite Hill, Teese

Yogurt: Silk, So Delicious Dairy Free, Stonyfield Farm O'Soy

Milk: Almond Breeze, Calafia, Dream, Earth Balance, Edensoy, Engine 2, Good Karma, Living Harvest Tempt, Organic Valley, Pacific, Silk, So Delicious Dairy Free, Westsoy

Creamer: Silk, So Delicious Dairy Free, Stonyfield Organic

Whipped cream: Soyatoo (soy and rice base)

Mock Meats

Chicken: Beyond Meat, Boca, Gardein, Match, Morningstar Farms*, Tofurky

Beef: Beyond Beef, Boca, Field Roast, Gardein, Match

Pork: Field Roast, Lightlife, Match, Yves

Seafood: Match, Sophie's Kitchen

---

*Morningstar Farms makes both vegan and vegetarian products. Check the package carefully for egg or milk ingredients.

<u>**Dressings and Sauces**</u>

Salad Dressing: Annie's Naturals, Bragg, OrganicVille

BBQ and Ketchup: Annie's BBQ, OrganicVille

Soy Sauces: Bragg Liquid Amino, Coconut Secret Raw Organic
Vegan Coconut Aminos (soy-free "Soy" sauce), San J Tamari
Soy Sauce

New vegan brands and products are popping up every day. It's an
exciting time to be a vegan!

Helpful Tips

Keep your fridge and pantry stocked. If you always have access to
healthy, delicious, vegan foods, you'll be more likely to stick to
your new eating plan.

Know what you like to eat. Do you love tempura-fried veggies or
have a special family recipe for beer-battered onion rings? Get
some Ener-G egg replacer to use as a binder in your batter. Do you
frequently prepare cream soups? Make sure you have non-dairy
milk on hand. Do you bring a BLT sandwich to work for lunch?
Hop over to the veggie "meat" aisle and pick up some soy bacon.
Once you know that you can make quick meals you love, it's a snap
to make the switch.

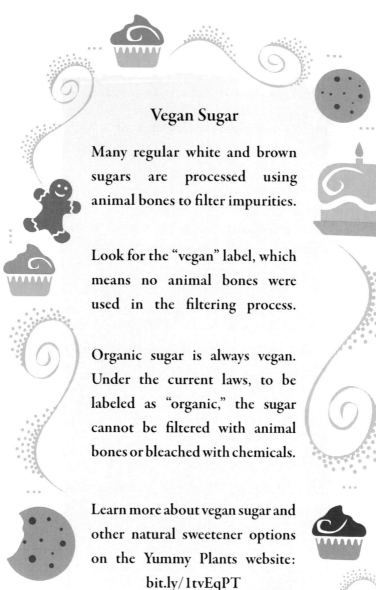

Vegan Sugar

Many regular white and brown sugars are processed using animal bones to filter impurities.

Look for the "vegan" label, which means no animal bones were used in the filtering process.

Organic sugar is always vegan. Under the current laws, to be labeled as "organic," the sugar cannot be filtered with animal bones or bleached with chemicals.

Learn more about vegan sugar and other natural sweetener options on the Yummy Plants website: bit.ly/1tvEqPT

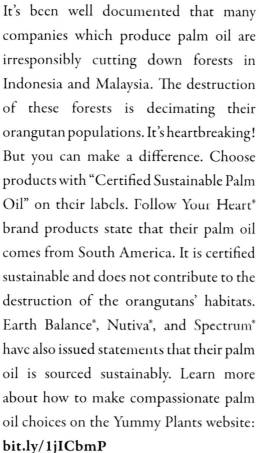

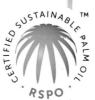

**Do you know about palm oil?
Learn how you can help!**

It's been well documented that many companies which produce palm oil are irresponsibly cutting down forests in Indonesia and Malaysia. The destruction of these forests is decimating their orangutan populations. It's heartbreaking! But you can make a difference. Choose products with "Certified Sustainable Palm Oil" on their labels. Follow Your Heart® brand products state that their palm oil comes from South America. It is certified sustainable and does not contribute to the destruction of the orangutans' habitats. Earth Balance®, Nutiva®, and Spectrum® have also issued statements that their palm oil is sourced sustainably. Learn more about how to make compassionate palm oil choices on the Yummy Plants website: **bit.ly/1jICbmP**

SAVE THE ORANGUTANS!

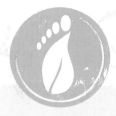

Reduce your carbon footprint, buy local.

Farmers' markets offer fresh, locally grown seasonal produce. You'll typically see more varieties of fruits and vegetables at the markets than you'll find at your local grocery store. Imagine zebra tomatoes, white carrots, and exotic greens. It's an adventure! Enter your zip code at Local Harvest to find farmers markets in your area.

localharvest.org/farmers-markets

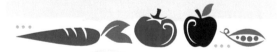

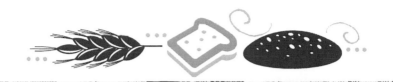

CHAPTER 3

Introduction to Grains and Seeds

Part of the fun of exploring vegan food is learning about all the textures and flavors of grains and the seeds we eat as grains. From amaranth to quinoa, to wheat, spelt, and rice, there is a huge variety of flavors, vitamins, and nutrients waiting for you to explore.

Gluten-free Grains

Amaranth is slightly sweet with very tiny grains. It becomes somewhat sticky when cooked. Be careful not to overcook it or it might become one really big amaranth clump. Amaranth is high in protein and calcium. It's a good source of magnesium, phosphorus, and iron.

Buckwheat has an earthy, nutty flavor, and isn't wheat at all. It's a seed we eat as a grain. Buckwheat is a good source of manganese, copper, and magnesium. It's delicious in crepes and pancakes.

Millet has a sweet flavor and is packed with protein. Another of the "ancient grains," millet has been used as a staple in Africa and India for thousands of years. It's also high in iron and rich in B vitamins.

Oats have a creamy texture and aren't just for breakfast. Oats are now being transformed into non-dairy milks! Whole-grain oats are a good source of soluble fiber. They have a low glycemic index, which means that blood sugar levels will remain more stable during the digestion process.

Quinoa, another seed we eat as a grain, can be sweet or savory depending on how it's prepared. It takes on the flavor of the base sauce or broth. Quinoa contains all of the essential amino acids and is a good source of fiber and iron.

Rice is a complex carbohydrate that's easily digestible and tolerated by most people. Nutritionists often call rice "the great balancer."

Grains Containing Gluten

Barley has a nutty flavor and a chewy texture. It is very high in soluble fiber and beneficial for the "friendly" bacteria in the large intestine. Barley contains eight of the nine essential amino acids. New studies find that eating whole barley may help regulate blood sugar.

Kamut® berries are about twice as large as traditional wheat berries and have a richer, nuttier flavor. It's one of the "ancient grains" and was originally cultivated thousands of years ago in Egypt. Kamut, actually a brand name for this variety of ancient wheat, has avoided the genetic modifications of our modern wheat. It may be eaten as whole berries or milled for use as flour.

Spelt is another variety of wheat and has the signature nutty flavor. It's commonly called one of the "ancient grains" and can be eaten as whole berries or milled for use as flour.

Wheat has a rich, nutty flavor and can be eaten as whole berries or milled for use as flour. Cooked wheatberries add a nice, chewy texture to a dish and are a good source of fiber.

Time-Saving Tips

Cook a few different grains on a weekend and store in the fridge. During the week, you can quickly reheat your grains and add some fresh cooked veggies to create a delicious and nutritious meal. It will take less than 15 minutes to sauté, steam, or roast most chopped vegetables. If you're really pressed for time, cook frozen vegetables in the microwave and add them to precooked grains.

See the chart on the following page for cook times per 1 cup of grains.

1. Measure the dry grain and rinse in cold water.

2. Drain grains and discard the soak water.

3. Add grains to water and bring to a boil.
   Reduce heat, cover and simmer.

All measurements and times are approximate. Keep an eye on your grains. Check at the halfway point to see if more liquid is needed. *Note:* If there is too much liquid, remove the lid and boil off the excess water.

Reheat cooked grain on the stove. Add a small amount of liquid to a pan and cook on low. Grains may also be reheated in the oven: bake at 300 °F for 10 to 15 minutes.

COOK TIME FOR GRAINS

1 CUP GRAINS	WATER	COOKING TIME
Amaranth	2-½ cups	20 minutes
Brown rice	2 cups	50 minutes
Barley (pearled)*	3 cups	40 minutes
Barley (hulled)	3 cups	1 hour
Buckwheat (kasha)	2 cups	20 minutes
Kamut*	3 cups	1-½ hours
Millet	2-3 cups	30 minutes
Oats (whole groats)	3 cups	30 minutes
Oatmeal (rolled oats)	2 cups	10 minutes
Quinoa	2 cups	20 minutes
Spelt*	3 cups	1-½ hours
Wheat berries*	2-3 cups	1-½ hours
Wild rice	2 cups	1 hour

* Soak overnight. Without soaking, double the cook time.

Change the texture of your grains!

Did you know you can change the texture of grains like quinoa, millet, and buckwheat with different cooking methods? Bring the liquid to a boil before adding your grains to keep them separate like rice. Start with cold water and boil your grains to create a softer, more porridge-like consistency.

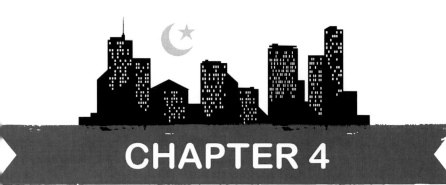

CHAPTER 4

Out and About – How to Stay Vegan

Sticking to your plant-based eating plan at office potlucks, bagel breakfast days, and offsite client meetings is as easy as vegan pie once you have a strategy.

Tips for the Office

Bring a plate of gooey, dairy-free chocolate-chip cookies or a savory main dish to share with your colleagues for potlucks to show them how delicious vegan food really is. (See Recipes, starting on page 51.) This positive approach allows you to enjoy communal dining situations and gives co-workers a chance to taste delicious vegan foods.

- 🍽 Keep shelf-stable non-dairy milk at your desk for impromptu team breakfasts.

- 🍽 Keep vegan butter and cream cheese in the fridge for office bagel days.

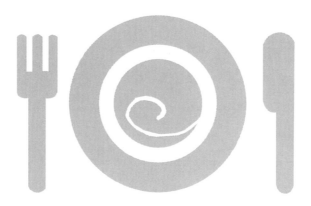

Tips for Client Meetings at Restaurants

There are many cuisines that naturally have an abundance of vegan options including Chinese, Ethiopian, Greek, Indian, Italian, Middle Eastern, Mexican, Thai, and Japanese. Double-check with your server to be sure your order is vegan. Sometimes meat and dairy are hidden in sauces and vegetable dishes.

- Greek: Confirm that the grape leaves and stuffed peppers are stuffed with rice (not meat).

- Indian: Confirm a dish is free of ghee or other dairy products.

- Italian: Confirm the pasta is egg-free.

- Mexican: Confirm the rice and beans are free of pork, chicken stock, or lard.

- Thai and Japanese: Confirm that the curries, noodles, and soups are fish-free.

If your client has picked a steakhouse or a seafood restaurant, call the restaurant in advance to ask about options for a meatless, eggless, dairy-free meal. (*Note:* This type of conversation with the chef works best at an off-time, such as 3:00 P.M. or 4:00 P.M. several days before the reservation.)

If there's no time to discuss vegan options with the chef, you'll still be fine. Salads, baked potatoes, cheese-free pizza, and pasta with marinara sauce are solid vegan choices at many mainstream eateries.

If you can choose the restaurant, it's worth scouting reviews from your local vegan meetup group to find the best veg-friendly hotspots.

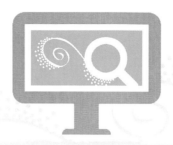

Search online for the best vegan-friendly eats:

 Happycow.net is a large restaurant database that focuses specifically on vegetarian and vegan restaurants.

 Yelp.com is one of the largest global restaurant databases for all types of food. Search for the keyword "vegan."

 Yummyplants.com is a vegan lifestyle website. View the database of vegan-friendly restaurants suggessted by our community members: **yummyplants.com/ vegan-friendly-restaurants/**

Out on the Town

Vegan happy hour snacks are available at many bars and restaurants. When you're out with your friends, try munching on:

- 🍽 Stacked nachos with beans, jalapenos, olives (hold the cheese)

- 🍽 Sushi rolls with avocado, cucumber, or shiitake mushrooms

- 🍽 Hummus and olive plate

- 🍽 Chips and guacamole

Lessons Learned from the French

In France, people meet for *apéro* hour, and cafes often serve olives, nuts, or salty crackers alongside those glasses of wine or Pastis. If you wanted to have a backup plan, carry a bag of shelled, salted peanuts for a fool-proof, French-style apéro hour, wherever you happen to be in the world.

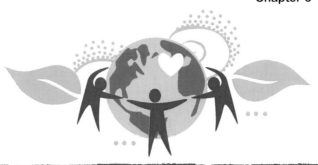

CHAPTER 5

Helpful Resources

Community

You're not alone! There are millions of people just like you, all over the world, exploring a plant-based lifestyle. Do you have questions about the yummiest vegan ice cream or which non-dairy cheese melts the best on pizza? There is a forum on the Yummy Plants website where you can ask questions about vegan products, restaurants, recipes... anything! Ask questions, get answers. Share what works for you. We're all working together in unity to help support each other. Post your question here: **bit.ly/1pI0x5e**

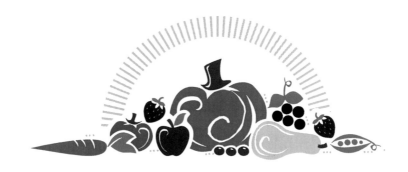

Health: Information That Supports a Vegan Diet

If your nearest and dearest are worried that your diet rich in phytonutrients, fiber, and great taste isn't supplying all the nutrients you need, allay their fears by letting them know that medical evidence supports a plant-based diet as a healthy diet. Ninety-nine percent of your calcium, protein, vitamins, and other nutritional needs can be met purely from plants. (See Vitamin B12 sidebar, page 27.) Have them browse **pcrm.org**, **nutitionfacts.org**, and **diseaseproof.com** for more information about the health benefits of a vegan diet.

Here are additional online resources from the health section of the Yummy Plants website:

Weight loss: Dr. Neal Barnard from PCRM discusses the effectiveness of a vegan meal plan to successfully overcome obesity.

bit.ly/1oIpXm3

Health benefits: Dr. Neal Barnard from PCRM discusses the health benefits of eating plant-based foods.

bit.ly/SmkIdz

Health promoting foods: Dr. Joel Fuhrman of Diseaseproof.com discusses the protective properties of specific nutrient-dense foods.

bit.ly/1kvbNNl

Calcium: Dr. Neal Barnard from PCRM discusses how to get enough calcium and keep it in our bones.

bit.ly/RRinXH

Dr. Joel Fuhrman of Diseaseproof.com discusses plant-based sources of calcium and support that a vegan diet can prevent osteoporosis.

bit.ly/1mEhjjr

CHAPTER 6

Sample Meals

Let's get cooking! Try a 1-week sample meal plan that incorporates familiar tasting transitional foods that take some of the mystery out of plant-based eating. Yogurt, ice cream, and pizza are included in the meal plan, along with lots of fresh fruits and vegetables.

All of the foods mentioned in this section are vegan. When "milk" or "meat" is mentioned, it's the fabulous faux version made from nuts, grains, and vegetable proteins. These plant-based foods are nutritious, delicious, and better for you and the environment than their more traditional counterparts. Have fun experimenting with tasty new versions of your favorite foods!

Breakfast

Day 1   Granola with milk

Day 2   Oatmeal with apples and cinnamon

Day 3   Yogurt topped with strawberries and walnuts

Day 4   Waffles topped with fruit

Day 5   Smoothie and toast with butter and jam

Day 6   Pancakes with maple syrup

Day 7   Bagel with cream cheese

Lunch

Day 1   Chili

Day 2   Grilled cheese and tomato sandwich

Day 3   Pizza bagel with salad

Day 4   Split pea soup and salad

Day 5   Rice and beans with tortillas, sour cream, cheese, and salsa

Day 6   Chicken salad

Day 7   BALT sandwich (bacon, avocado, lettuce, and tomato)

Dinner entrées

Day 1   Mac and cheese served with green beans

Day 2   Pasta with tomato sauce served with vegetable soup

Day 3   Veggie burgers served with roasted potatoes

Day 4   Mushroom pizza served with steamed asparagus

Day 5   Rice pilaf served with broccoli soup

Day 6   Meatloaf with mashed potatoes and gravy

Day 7   Portabella mushrooms sautéed with broccoli, potatoes, and peas over rice

Recipes

Start off with this collection of quick and easy vegan recipes for breakfast, lunch, snacks, dinner, and dessert. For more vegan recipes, browse the entire recipe database at **yummyplants.com/all-vegan-recipes/**

Note: If a recipe calls for vegetable broth, it can be made quickly with water and bouillon cubes.

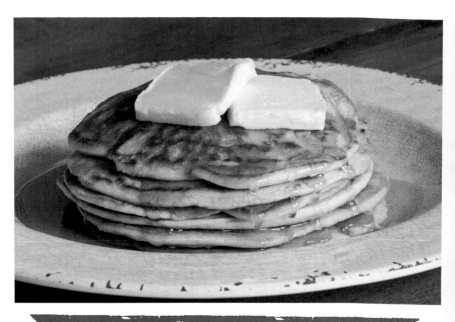

Pancakes with Maple Syrup (page 56)

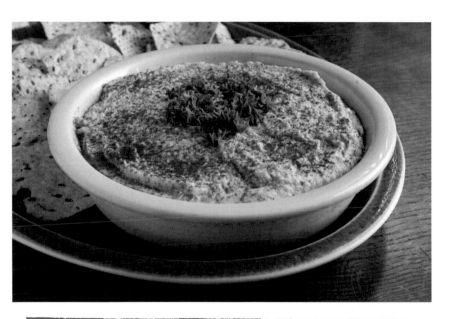

Hummus (page 75)

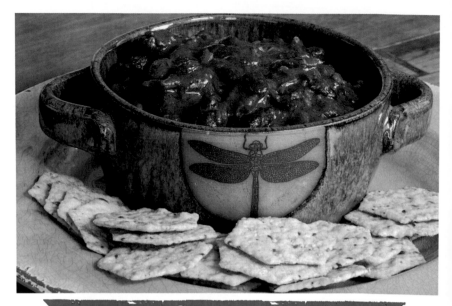

Chili (page 66)

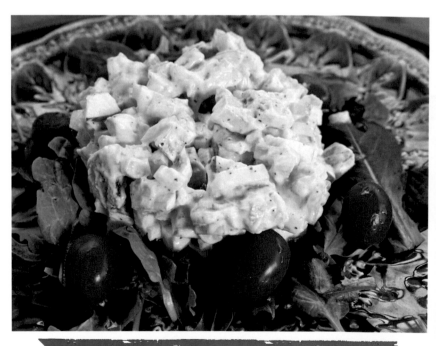

No Chicken Salad (page 68)

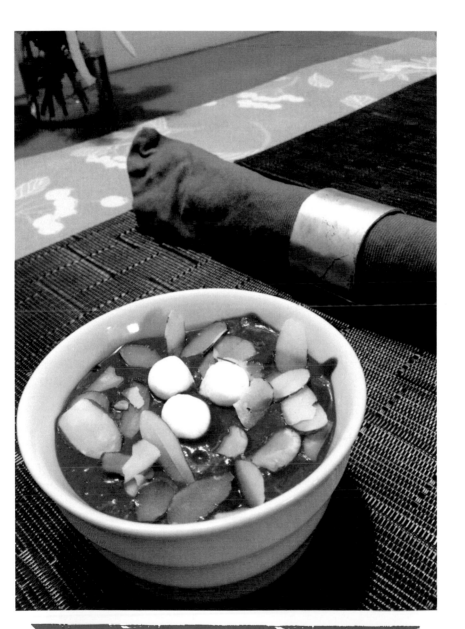

S'mores Pudding (page 83)

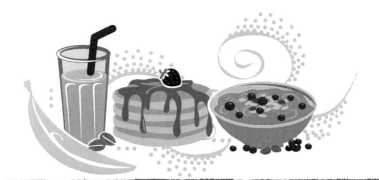

BREAKFAST RECIPES

Baked Oatmeal

Prep time = 2 minutes, Cook time = 45 minutes, Servings = 8

Makes a bunch: perfect for weekend brunch with friends.

2 cups rolled oats

2 cups non-dairy milk

½ cup walnut pieces

⅓ cup maple syrup

1 teaspoon baking powder

1½ teaspoons ground cinnamon

½ teaspoon salt

1½ teaspoons of Ener-G egg replacer plus 2 tablespoons of water

3 tablespoons of butter, melted

2 teaspoons vanilla extract

2 ripe bananas, cut into ½-inch pieces

1½ cups blueberries

1. Preheat the oven to 375 °F. Grease the inside of an 8-inch square baking dish. Dissolve the Ener-G egg replacer in 2 tablespoons of water and set aside.

2. In a bowl, mix the dry ingredients together: the oats, half the walnuts, baking powder, cinnamon, and salt.

3. In another bowl, whisk together the wet ingredients: the maple syrup, non-dairy milk, vanilla, half the butter, and the Ener-G egg replacer mixture.

4. Place the sliced bananas in a single layer in the bottom of the greased baking dish. Sprinkle two-thirds of the berries on top of the bananas. Cover the fruit with the dry oat mixture. Slowly drizzle the wet mixture over the oats. Gently shake the baking dish to make sure the liquid moves throughout all the oats. Sprinkle the remaining berries and walnuts on top.

5. Bake for 35 to 45 minutes until the top is golden brown. Remove from the oven and let cool for a few minutes. Drizzle the remaining butter on top and serve.

Blueberry Quinoa with Coconut Milk

Prep time = 1 minute, Cook time = 25 minutes, Servings = 2

A delicious hot breakfast treat on a cold morning.
Let it simmer while you're getting ready for work or school.

½ cup quinoa

1 cup water

¼ cup of fresh blueberries

Maple syrup

Unsweetened coconut milk
(So Delicious® Dairy Free
works well)

1. Place the quinoa, water, and blueberries in a pot. Cover the pot and bring to a boil. Reduce heat to simmer and cook for another 20 minutes, stirring occasionally. As some of the blueberries disintegrate, the quinoa will turn a slightly purplish color.

2. Once the water has been absorbed, serve in individual bowls. Top with maple syrup and add coconut milk or creamer to taste.

Pancakes with Maple Syrup

Prep time = 5 minutes, Cook time = 5 minutes per pancake, Servings = 8

A fresh, hot breakfast to start your day with a smile.

1 cup flour	⅛ teaspoon salt
1 tablespoon maple syrup	1 cup non-dairy milk
2 tablespoons baking powder	2 tablespoons vegetable oil

1. Combine the flour, baking powder, and salt in a large bowl. Stir in the milk, maple syrup, and oil until batter is smooth.

2. Drop ¼ cup of batter at a time onto a hot, oiled griddle over medium high heat. When bubbles appear on the surface of the pancake (after approximately 3 minutes), it's time to flip. Cook the other side for another 2 minutes.

Sundae Smoothie

Prep time = 1 minute, Cook time = 1 minute, Servings = 2

It's a liquid sundae that's packed with Vitamin C.
For a raw option, make your own nut milk. (See page 18.)

1 ½ cups of unsweetened non-dairy milk

1 packet of frozen açai purée (unsweetened)

2 tablespoons cocoa powder

¼ cup of walnuts

1 large ripe banana

Add all ingredients to your blender. Blend until smooth.

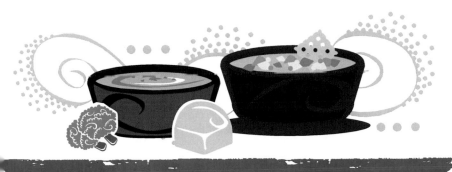

SOUPS AND SAUCES

Cream of Broccoli Soup

Prep time = 15 minutes, Cook time = 30 minutes, Servings = 6

Healthy tastes delicious. This recipe uses four cups of broccoli. It reheats well and can be made the day before company arrives.

4 cups broccoli, chopped	2 small potatoes, chopped
1 cup broccoli florets (for garnish)	2 cups unsweetened non-dairy milk
½ cup dried shiitake mushrooms soaked in 1 cup of warm water	2 cups vegetable broth
	1 teaspoon salt
	1 teaspoon pepper

1. Soak ½ cup of dried shiitake mushrooms in 1 cup of hot water. Soak for 15 minutes. Set aside.

2. Chop 4 cups of broccoli plus 1 cup of broccoli florets for garnish. Steam the broccoli for 5-10 minutes, or until tender.

3. While steaming the broccoli, add two cups of vegetable broth, potatoes, salt, and pepper to a large pot. Add shiitake mushrooms and soak liquid. Cook for about 10 minutes, or until tender.

4. Once the potatoes are cooked, transfer entire contents of the pot to your blender. Purée until completely liquefied and pour back into the pot.

5. Place half of the steamed broccoli in the blender along with the milk. Purée broccoli until liquefied and pour into pot.

6. Place the remaining broccoli in the blender with enough soup liquid to cover. Pulse until desired consistency is reached.

7. Transfer broccoli mixture to the pot and stir well. Simmer for about 5 minutes. Serve in individual bowls and garnish with broccoli florets.

Video link: Watch this recipe being made on TV!
▶ **cbsloc.al/1ufOVZZ**

Roasted Squash Soup

Prep time = 30 minutes, Cook time = 1 hour, Servings = 6

Decadently rich and creamy, this soup is deeply satisfying.

3 pounds of butternut squash
4 cups of vegetable broth
1 teaspoon dried thyme
1 teaspoon dried sage
Parsley for garnish
Salt and pepper to taste

Nut cream
1 cup of raw, unsalted cashews
1 cup of vegetable broth

1. Preheat oven to 400 °F.

2. Cut squash in half and remove seeds. Place on a baking sheet (cut-side down) and bake 30-40 minutes until tender.

3. While squash is roasting, prepare the nut cream. Add nuts to blender with ½ cup of vegetable broth. Pulse slowly to mix. Then add the remaining ½ cup of broth and process until mixture is smooth and creamy. Set cream aside.

4. Once the squash is cooked, remove skin, cut into small pieces, and transfer to a large soup pot. Add 4 cups of vegetable broth and dried spices. Bring mixture to a boil, then turn down the heat and simmer for 20 minutes, covered.

5. Transfer soup to blender. Don't fill blender all the way to the top as the liquid will be very hot. Process in small batches and blend until smooth.

6. Return the blended soup to the pot and stir in the nut cream, reserving ¼ cup of the cream as garnish. Add salt and pepper to taste.

7. Serve soup in bowls. Drizzle the remaining nut cream on top and garnish with parsley.

Split Pea Soup

Prep time = 15 minutes, Cook time = 75 minutes, Servings = 6

A thick and hearty soup that's simple to prepare.

1½ cups quick-cooking
  split peas

6 cups of vegetable broth

⅔ cup onion, chopped

¾ cup carrot, chopped

½ cup celery, chopped

½ teaspoon dried parsley

1 bay leaf

¼ teaspoon dried thyme

Salt to taste

Pepper to taste

1. Rinse peas. Combine split peas and vegetable broth in a large pot. Bring to a boil, cover pot, and simmer for 45 minutes, until peas are tender.

2. Add vegetables and seasonings (except salt and pepper). Cook on low, covered, an additional 15 minutes, adding water if mixture is too thick.

3. Remove from heat. Remove bay leaf. Transfer soup to a blender and process until desired consistency is reached. Transfer soup to a large bowl. Add salt and pepper to taste. Ladle into small bowls and serve.

Vegetable Soup

Prep time = 15 minutes, Cook time = 30 minutes, Servings = 6

A delicious staple to keep stocked in your fridge.

3 tablespoons olive oil	¼ teaspoon dried parsley
¼ onion, diced	¼ teaspoon sugar
2 carrots, chopped	2 tomatoes, diced
2 stalks of celery, chopped	2 small potatoes, diced
6 cups of vegetable broth	½ cup frozen peas
1 large bay leaf	Salt to taste
1 teaspoon dried thyme	Pepper to taste

1. Heat the olive oil in a medium saucepan. Add onion, carrots, and celery. Cover the saucepan and cook the vegetables on a low heat for 5 minutes, until the onions are brown. Stir frequently.

2. Add vegetable broth and spices (except for salt and pepper). Bring to a boil. Add the tomatoes, potatoes, and sugar. Cover the pan and allow the mixture to simmer for 25 minutes.

3. After 20 minutes, taste for seasoning. Add frozen vegetables. Add salt and pepper to taste. Continue cooking until the frozen vegetables are done. Serve immediately or store in refrigerator until needed.

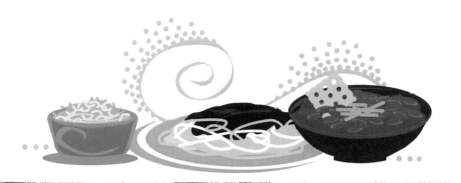

ENTRÉES

Chili

Prep time = 20 minutes, Cook time = 20 minutes, Servings = 4

Chili is quick to prepare and stores well for next-day lunches. Serve with crackers or over rice.

Optional: Add a "meaty" texture with a faux beef product. Melt some vegan cheese on top.

½ yellow onion, diced

1 clove garlic, minced

½ large bell pepper, diced

1 tablespoon red pepper flakes (optional)

1 teaspoon cumin

14 oz. of diced tomatoes

2 tablespoons of tomato paste

1 teaspoon of oil

15 oz. can of kidney or pinto beans

1 cup of water

Salt and pepper to taste

Optional: 1 package of faux beef (Beyond Meat® Beefy Crumbles works well)

Optional: top with vegan cheese (Follow Your Heart® melts well)

1. Heat 3 tablespoons of oil or water in a medium-sized sauce pot. Add the onions and garlic. Sauté on a low-medium heat until soft, about 10 minutes.

2. Add all spices and optional vegan beef. Cook for 2 minutes.

3. Add tomato paste and crushed tomatoes, kidney beans, and cup of water. Stir until well combined. Bring to a boil, then simmer for 10 minutes or until desired thickness is reached. Add salt and pepper to taste. Optional: Top with vegan cheese.

Mac and Cheese

Prep time = 5 minutes, Cook time = 15 minutes, Servings = 4

Enjoy a delicious new version of a childhood favorite.
The cheese sauce also makes a rich and creamy topping
for broccoli, asparagus, potatoes, and other vegetables.

12 ounces dry macaroni

1½ cups unsweetened non-dairy milk

¾ cup nutritional yeast

1 teaspoon stone ground mustard

½ teaspoon salt

½ teaspoon pepper

½ teaspoon curry powder

¼ teaspoon garlic powder

Parsley, chopped for garnish

Optional: Steamed broccoli crowns

1. Cook the macaroni according to instructions.

2. While the macaroni is cooking, add all of the sauce ingredients to a pot and mix well. Cook over medium heat and bring sauce to a boil. Reduce heat to simmer and cook for about five minutes, stirring occasionally, until the sauce starts to thicken. When sauce reaches desired consistency, remove from heat. If sauce gets too thick, add more milk.

3. Transfer macaroni to a serving bowl. Pour cheese sauce over macaroni. Add optional broccoli crowns. Garnish with parsley.

No Chicken Salad

Prep time = 5 minutes, Cook time = 3 minutes, Servings = 4

No Chicken Salad makes an excellent portable meal. It's a delicious filling for pita pockets and lunch box sandwiches. It also works well as a salad topping.

1½ cups diced celery

1½ cups chopped apple

1 cup vegan mayonnaise

Pinch of salt

½ teaspoon pepper

2 tablespoons lemon juice

3 cups cooked vegan chicken, chopped (Beyond Meat, lightly seasoned flavor works well)

Chopped parsley for garnish

1. In a large bowl, toss chicken with diced celery, apples, and mayonnaise. Mix well.

2. Add lemon juice, salt and pepper to taste. Garnish with parsley.

3. Make pita sandwiches or plate individually on a bed of mixed greens with tomatoes.

Watch the video and learn how to make No Chicken Salad!
▶ bit.ly/1kB5bC6

Pasta with Creamy Tomato Sauce

Prep time = 20 minutes, Cook time = 40 minutes,
Servings = 6-8 (approximately 4 cups of sauce)

*The secret to the creamy texture is to purée all the vegetables.
Try making it with locally grown summer tomatoes for an
extra rich sauce.*

3 tablespoons olive oil

1 large onion, chopped

½ large green pepper, chopped

½ carrot, chopped

1 small garlic clove, chopped

4 cups tomatoes, chopped

1 large bay leaf

8 sprigs of fresh parsley, chopped

1 sprig of thyme, chopped

3 fresh basil leaves, chopped

¼ teaspoon salt

Dash of pepper

½ teaspoon of sugar

1 pound of pasta*

1. Heat olive oil in a medium saucepan. Add onion, green pepper, garlic, and carrot. Cook over medium heat until onion is brown, stirring frequently. Add tomatoes, bay leaf, parsley, thyme, salt, and pepper. Bring mixture to a boil then simmer covered for 35 minutes, stirring occasionally.

2. Add sugar. Cook for 3 minutes more. Remove the bay leaf. Let sauce cool for several minutes.

3. Cook pasta according to instructions. While pasta is cooking, put the sauce in the blender and blend until smooth.

4. Rinse and drain cooked pasta. Plate individually, top with sauce, and garnish with fresh parsley.

* Make sure the pasta is egg-free.

Quinoa Pilaf

Prep time = 5 minutes, Cook time = 30 minutes, Servings = 4

This protein-packed recipe stores well for several days in the refrigerator.

1½ tablespoons olive oil
1 cup quinoa
2 cups vegetable broth
1 bell pepper, chopped
½ cup onion, chopped

½ cup walnuts or almonds, chopped
Parsley for garnish
Salt to taste
Pepper to taste

1. Heat oil in a pot over medium-high heat. Add onion and cook for about 5 minutes, until translucent.

2. Add vegetables and cook the mixture an additional 3 minutes.

3. Add quinoa and broth to the saucepan. Bring mixture to a boil. Cover the pot and reduce heat to simmer. Simmer 15 to 20 minutes until the quinoa is soft and fluffy.

4. Remove from heat. Add nuts and mix well. Plate individually and garnish with parsley.

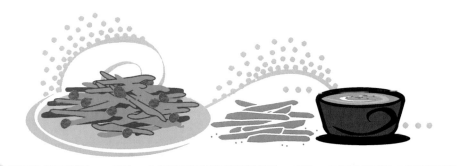

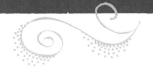

SIDES AND SNACKS

Candied Yams

Prep time = 15 minutes, Cook time = 1 hour 10 minutes, Servings = 12

Candied yams add a sweet treat to any meal.

10 medium yams, peeled and sliced	1 cup light brown sugar
½ cup vegan butter	½ cup water
¾ teaspoon salt	1 teaspoon vanilla flavoring
	¾ cup pecans, chopped

1. Cover yams with water. Bring water to boil then simmer yams for about 50 - 60 minutes, until tender.

2. While the yams are cooking, prepare the sauce. Add butter, salt, sugar, vanilla, and ½ cup water to a large pot. Stir over low heat until sugar dissolves. Bring to boil and cook 3 minutes, uncovered. Reduce heat to simmer.

3. Transfer yams to the pot. Stir in pecans. Heat uncovered for about 10 minutes. Transfer to a large bowl and serve.

Crispy Roasted Potatoes

Prep time = 5 minutes, Cook time = 30 minutes, Servings = 4

A healthier version of an American favorite.

4 potatoes, peeled and cubed   ⅛ teaspoon pepper
⅛ cup olive oil   ⅛ teaspoon dried parsley
⅛ teaspoon salt

1.   Preheat the oven to 425 °F. Line baking sheet with tin foil or a silicone mat.

2.   Mix salt, pepper, parsley, and oil together in a bowl. Add potatoes to the bowl and mix well until all are coated with oil.

3.   Place potatoes in a single layer on baking sheet. Bake at 425 °F for 20 minutes. Remove from oven, flip potatoes with spatula, and bake for 10 more minutes or until done. Potatoes should be crispy brown on edges when done.

Green Beans with Almonds

Prep time = 5 minutes, Cook time = 1 minute, Servings = 6

A quick and easy party dish that everyone will love.

½ cup vegan butter   Salt to taste
½ cup toasted almonds, sliced   Pepper to taste
1 pound of cooked green beans

1. Melt the butter in a frying pan. Add the almonds and brown for a minute.

2. Add the cooked green beans and heat until warm. Add salt and pepper to taste.

Hummus

Prep time = 5 minutes, Cook time = 5 minutes,
Servings = 3.75 cups

Hummus is a delicious plant-based protein source. It's fast, easy, and can stay in the fridge for a week. This recipe has 36 grams of protein from the garbanzo beans (18g per can).

2 cans of garbanzo beans
   (one drained, one with liquid)
¼ cup raw sesame seeds
1 tablespoon olive oil
¼ cup fresh lemon juice

½ teaspoon salt
1 teaspoon cumin
Smoked paprika and
parsley for garnish
Optional: 1 clove of garlic

1. Place all of the ingredients except the paprika and parsley into the blender. Blend for several minutes until creamy. You may need to stop the blender and scrape the sides to ensure even processing.

2. Transfer to a serving dish. Top with smoked paprika and chopped parsley.

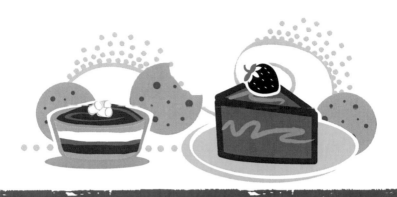

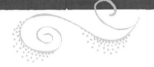

DESSERTS

Apple Compote

Prep time = 15 min, Cook time = 45 min, Servings = 3

Try topping with vegan ice cream.

2 large apples, peeled and sliced

1 cup apple juice

¾ cup breadcrumbs

1½ tablespoons ground cinnamon

½ cup sugar

1½ tablespoons vegan butter

1. Preheat the oven to 425 °F. Coat a small baking dish with non-stick spray.

2. Place a layer of apples on the bottom of the baking dish. Sprinkle a small amount of the cinnamon, sugar, and breadcrumbs onto apples. Add a second layer of sliced apples. Sprinkle with cinnamon, sugar, and breadcrumbs. Continue this process until all the apple slices are in the baking dish. Pour the apple juice and any remaining ingredients over the apples. Top with vegan butter.

3. Bake for 45 minutes or until apples are browned and soft. Serve warm.

Caramels

Prep time = 5 min, Cook time = 35 – 40 min,
Servings = Approximately 50 pieces

Chef's note: A candy thermometer is helpful for this recipe.

1 cup vegan butter	1 cup light corn syrup
2 cups sugar	3 teaspoons vanilla
2 cups non-dairy milk	

1. Line an 8.5 x 11-inch baking pan with parchment paper.

2. Add all ingredients except vanilla to a large pot. Make sure there is room to stir without liquid splashing outside the pot.

3. Cook over medium heat and bring ingredients to a boil, stirring frequently. Cook the mixture down to about ¼ of its original volume. It will take about 35 minutes.

4. Continue to cook over medium heat until mixture reaches 245 °F. Measure the temperature with a candy thermometer or test using a glass of cold water. Drip mixture from a spoon into a glass of cold water. When mixture makes a firm ball in the water, the candy is ready.

5. Remove from heat and allow to cool for 1-2 minutes. Stir in vanilla and pour into baking pan.

6. Allow to cool completely. Once the caramel has hardened, snip into cubes using kitchen shears or a very sharp knife. Wrap cubes individually with plastic wrap or place in mini cupcake holders.

Note: To make caramel sauce, heat to 230 °F and remove from heat. Let mixture stand for 1-2 minutes before adding the vanilla. Serve immediately or store in a glass jar. Keep refrigerated.

Chocolate Cake

Prep time = 10 min, Cook time = 30 min, Servings = 8

Perfect for birthdays or a sweet treat. Top with ready-made vegan frosting, such as Cherrybrook vanilla frosting, or garnish with fruit.

1½ cups all-purpose flour

1 cup sugar

⅓ cup cocoa

⅓ cup vegetable oil

2 tablespoons apple cider vinegar

1 teaspoon vanilla

1 teaspoon baking soda

½ teaspoon salt

1 cup cold water

1. Preheat the oven to 350 °F. In a large bowl, combine the dry ingredients: flour, sugar, cocoa, baking soda, and salt.

2. Make a small hole in the middle and gradually add in the wet ingredients: oil, vinegar, vanilla, and water. Stir the mixture with a slotted spoon or fork until well combined. Transfer to a 9-inch round cake pan and bake for 30 minutes.

3. Remove from oven and test to make sure it's fully cooked. Poke a toothpick into the center of the cake. If toothpick comes out clean, the cake is done. Otherwise, bake for 5 more minutes and test again. Repeat the process until the toothpick comes out clean.

4. Once cooked, let cake cool for 10 minutes before removing from the pan. Then cut around the outside edge of the cake with a sharp knife. Turn pan over onto a plate, let cool for another 10 minutes, and slice cake.

Chocolate Chip Cookies

Prep time = 15 minutes, Cook time = 15 minutes,
Servings = 20 cookies

Easy to make, delightful to eat. Since there are no eggs, the dough can be eaten raw!

Note: You'll need two non-stick baking sheets plus a wire rack to cool the cookies.

⅓ cup soy milk
1 tablespoon flaxseed, ground
½ teaspoon apple cider vinegar
⅓ cup vegan butter, softened
1 cup sugar

1 teaspoon vanilla extract
1¾ cups flour
½ teaspoon baking soda
½ teaspoon salt
1 cup vegan chocolate chips

1. Preheat the oven to 375 °F. Mix soy milk, flax seed, and vinegar together in a small bowl. The mixture will thicken. Set aside.

2. Sift flour, baking soda, and salt together into a medium bowl.

3. In a large bowl or mixer, cream sugar and butter until fluffy. Add vanilla and the flax seed mixture. Combine thoroughly.

4. Add the dry ingredients, stirring until well combined. Mix in the chocolate chips.

5. Drop spoonfuls of dough onto the cookie sheet, about 1 inch apart. Bake for 10-14 minutes. Check after 10 minutes.

6. When cookies are golden on top, remove from oven. Let sit 2-3 minutes on the cookie sheet, then transfer to a wire rack to cool completely.

Note: Sunspire 60% organic dark chocolate chips are vegan.

Drunken Prunes

Prep time = 5 minutes, Cook time = 24 hours, Servings = 24

A wonderful gift for the holidays – or any time you need to bring a hostess gift.

1 package dried prunes	1 bar dark chocolate
1 package raw almonds	1 cup dark rum or cognac

1. Soak prunes and almonds in a dish of rum or cognac overnight.

2. After soaking, remove the pits from the prunes. Place almonds inside the prunes (replacing the pits).

3. Melt chocolate in a double boiler. Be carful not to get any water in the chocolate, or you may get lumps. (It will still taste delicious, but it won't look as nice.)

4. Use a fork or chopsticks to dip prunes in the melted chocolate. Place on top of toothpicks or on a wire rack to cool.

5. Cool for about 20 minutes, then transfer to mini cupcake wrappers and refrigerate (about 2 hours) until the chocolate is hard.

S'mores Pudding

Prep time = 5 min, Cook time = 2 min, Servings = 2

A quick dessert that's elegant for company.

Note: If you can't find vegan marshmallows in your area, you can buy Sweet and Sara through her website or Dandies vegan marshmallows online through Amazon.

2 medium frozen bananas

3 tablespoons cocoa powder

4 tablespoons unsweetened non-dairy milk

½ cup mini vegan marshmallows

3 graham crackers

Sliced almonds for topping

1. Add frozen bananas to blender. Pulse and slowly add milk. Minimal processing is best.

2. Add cocoa powder, graham crackers, and ½ cup of marshmallows. Continue to pulse until mixture has the desired consistency, chunky or smooth.

3. Transfer mixture into serving dish and top with sliced almonds and mini-marshmallows. Chill for 1 hour before serving.

END NOTES

Start Eating Vegan Today!

Now you have all the information you need to easily start eating vegan. You've learned about easy food substitutions, you've got some basic recipes, and you even have a community support system where you can ask questions. The next step is to put your new knowledge into practice!

If you want to ease your way in, take baby steps. Begin by swapping out dairy milk in your morning coffee and replacing it with a rich soy creamer. When you're ready for the next step, top your bagels with vegan butter or cream cheese. You'll find that these changes are easy and you enjoy what you're eating. As your taste buds change, it becomes easier and easier to make more substitutions.

If you're ready to jump right in, head to the grocery store and make the swaps all at once.

Pick up some transitional convenience foods like sandwich slices, vegan cheeses, and non-dairy milks, and load up on the fresh fruit, veggies, and whole grains that will form the cornerstones of many delicious vegan meals. In about three weeks, you will have adjusted to the dietary changes. Dr. Neal Barnard of the Physicians Committee for Responsible Medicine says, "Twenty-one days is a magic number for changing any sort of habit. Two days doesn't give a person enough momentum and one year sounds daunting. Twenty-one days is enough time to break old habits and start on a new path."

Fast or slow, you can do this. Remember that help is available. When you tap into the Yummy Plants community of vegans all around the world, you'll find that you're part of one large family on a fun new adventure.

It really is easy to start eating vegan. I wish you radiant health, an abundance of energy, and all good things!

APPENDIX

BEANS AND LEGUMES

Approximate protein per cup (cooked)

Soybeans	29g
Lentils	18g
Adzuki beans	17g
Split peas	16g
Black beans	15g
Chickpeas	15g
Great northern beans	15g
Kidney beans	15g
Lima beans	15g
Navy beans	15g
Pinto beans	15g
Fava beans	14g
Mung beans	14g

GRAINS

Approximate protein per cup (cooked)

Kamut	11g
Spelt	11g
Amaranth	9g
Quinoa	8g
Wheat	7g
Wild rice	7g
Buckwheat	6g
Millet	6g
Oats	6g
Brown rice	5g
Barley	4g
White rice	4g

FRUITS AND VEGETABLES

All plants have some protein.
Approx. protein per 3.5 oz serving.

Apple	<1g	Honeydew	1g
Asparagus	4g	Kale	2g
Avocado	3g	Kiwi	2g
Bananas	2g	Lettuce	.5g
Bok choy	3g	Mushrooms (crimini)	2g
Broccoli	4g	Mustard greens	4g
Brussels sprouts	4g	Onion	2g
Cabbage	2g	Orange	2g
Cantaloupe	1g	Peppers	3g
Cauliflower	2g	Pineapple	1g
Celery	1g	Potato	3g
Cherries	2g	Radish	1g
Collard greens	5g	Spinach	5g
Dates	4g	Summer squash	2g
Eggplant	1g	Swiss chard	3g
Grapefruit	2g	Tomatoes	2g
Grapes	1g	Turnip greens	2g
Green beans	2g	Watermelon	1g
Green peas	7g	Yam	2g

INDEX

ACKNOWLEDGMENTS

There are so many people to thank. This project really did take a village! I want to acknowledge everyone who helped in ways large and small.

Aurelia d'Andrea, my amazing editor, read and edited each draft of this book with saintly patience. Ines Hubler, Kathrin Gassei, and Kristin Schroeder were my personal cheerleaders who encouraged me to finish writing the book.

Anita Barrett, Jennifer Kambas, and Marcy Smith, fabulous ladies with whom I have worked for many years, helped bring my vision into reality by creating a joyful, beautiful layout printed on earth-friendly paper. Keys Innovative Solutions, an RR Donnelley company, helped me navigate the world of print and find a way to make this project possible.

I so enjoyed connecting with family far and wide for this project. Bruce Gilbert resolved all contract and IP issues, Sara Gilbert edited and formatted the very first draft, and Ross Levin shaped the sample meal plan and stock your pantry sections.

Greg Stratton and Neeti Newaskar Attwood shared their culinary talents and photography skills to help with the recipes section. Colleen Cavolo, Julia Pamies Jassans, Juan Lopez, Meg Frattare, Chelsea Bugielski, Sushma Patel Bould, Karen Pisano, Katie Smallwood, Roots Market, Great Sage, Jana Savelkova, Jara Savelkova, Stephanie Hauskrecht, Milos Hauskrecht, and Alex Hauskrecht all helped with videos and photos for the book. Matthias Eck. Joy Zhang, and Ed Yaffa shared their technology know-how.

A special group of vegan chefs and cookbook authors advised and encouraged me: Jenny Engel, Heather Goldberg, Ellen Jaffe Jones, Brian Patton, and Laura Theodore.

Vegan bodybuilders Robert Cheeke and Derek Tresize helped create the video about vegan protein sources. Dr. Neal Barnard and Dr. Joel Fuhrman generously shared vegan health information with the Yummy Plants website. Their health tips are referenced on the resources page.

Vegan companies including Beyond Meat®, Follow Your Heart®, and So Delicious® Dairy Free, got on board immediately and donated coupons to help our readers sample new vegan products at a discount.

Finally, I want to thank my Mom, Shandel Gilbert, for her help both inside and outside of the kitchen.

Are you looking for more information about a vegan lifestyle? Visit the Yummy Plants website where we celebrate and share the joy of vegan food. Browse vegan recipes, product reviews, travel tips, videos, and more!

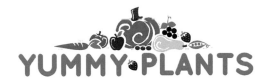

http://yummyplants.com

https://www.facebook.com/yummyplants

https://twitter.com/yummyplants

https://www.youtube.com/user/YummyPlants

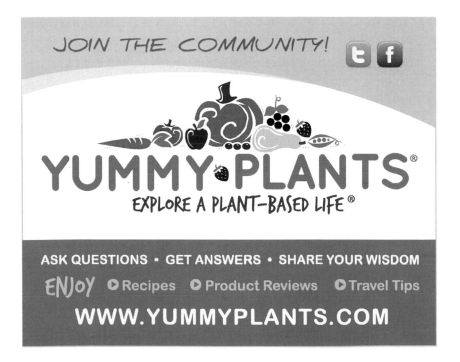

NOTES

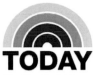

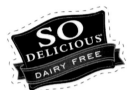

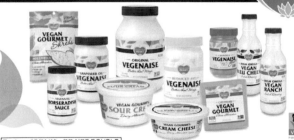